AF614044

"As someone who has been recently diagnosed with MS, I have been trying to learn everything about the disease and its treatment. This book has been so helpful to me and really fills a void in the literature by providing a first person account that presents many alternative therapies and advice. To hear this information first hand from someone else afflicted with MS is very comforting, and I will use this as a reference for years to come. It can be a very useful resource for people in all stages of the disease, especially in terms of providing beneficial ideas for therapies and treatments that you will most likely not learn about in the neurologist's office. There is even a chapter about knowing your rights in the workplace."

--TS

Multiple sclerosis patient

Treating Multiple Sclerosis

An Integrative Approach
You Will Not Get from
Your Doctor

REENA ARORA

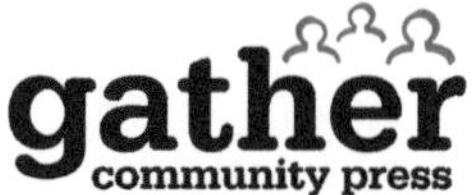

Gather Community Press
99 Summer Street, 7th Floor
Boston, MA 02110
(877) 775-7558

First published by Gather Community Press 12/8/2008

ISBN: 978-1-9350-2803-1 (sc)
ISBN: 978-1-9350-2804-8 (hc)

Library of Congress Control Number: 2008910195

Printed in the United States of America
Boston, Massachusetts

This book is printed on acid-free paper.

Dearest Mom and Dad,

Your courage is my inspiration, your support is my foundation, your falling tears are my falling tears, your wisdom is my strength and your strength leaves me speechless. Being your daughter is my blessing and I am so honored to voyage through life in the shelter of your love.

Love,

Me

TABLE OF CONTENTS

INTRODUCTION

Miserable that you have multiple sclerosis? Want to feel steady on your feet? Want some relief from the pain, dizziness, numbness, and disability? Well, I don't want to stop at just relief. I am determined to fix it. You may laugh and think, "Right…sure, lady!" but I decided that even if I walk down my path of fixing it and I fall short, at least I will make progress and find powerful tools along the way. This path has led me to managing my multiple sclerosis through lifestyle changes, allopathic medicine, homeopathic medicine, Ayurvedic medicine and dietary changes, all creating a holistic approach to my health management and resulting in relief from essentially all of my multiple sclerosis symptoms.

I am not a physician, so do not read this information as medical advice. Be sure to discuss any changes you wish to make in your health management with your physician. When I discuss alternative health care topics with my allopathic physicians, it is typically received with hesitation and caution, as is appropriate for the construct of western medical practice. However, I choose to continue with my pursuit and keep my physicians informed of my findings. Therefore, I am not well known as a compliant or cooperative patient to my health care providers, but I am conscientious about keeping them posted on what I am doing with treatments that do not fall under their area of expertise. I have gone from being a pain in the ass patient to a miracle patient, which makes it all worth it. I have endless gratitude for my allopathic health care providers for their skill, patience and forgiveness of my renegade defiant nature as a patient.

My educational background is in genetics and molecular biology. I received a Bachelors of Science in Genetics from the University of

Wisconsin – Madison and am currently enrolled in a graduate program in Cellular and Molecular Biology at the Illinois Institute of Technology. I also spent many years working as a scientist at Abbott Laboratories and in academic research and development environments. My understanding of genetics, cellular and molecular biology has enabled my inquiry into the molecular mechanisms of the remedies provided by western and eastern medicines.

A few years prior to my M.S. diagnosis, I was diagnosed with a kidney disease called focal segmental glomerulosclerosis. The very first prescription my nephrologists wrote for me was for a book entitled, *Remarkable Recovery* by C. Hirschberg, M.D. and M.I. Barasch, M.D., which is an evaluation and discussion of cases of stage four cancer patients who achieved spontaneous remissions.[1] The authors asked if these cases were really miracle cures, or did these

---

[1] Hirshberg, C. & Barasch, M. I. Remarkable Recovery. Riverhead Books, published by the Berkley Publishing Group, New York, NY. (1995).

patients have something in common that provided a platform for spontaneous remission of their cancers? They found that these patients were above all determined to cure themselves and did not accept the prognosis handed down by their physicians. The patients set out on their own individual journeys, mostly on unconventional paths, and through sheer determination, cured themselves of their cancers. Well gosh darnit! If they can do it with cancer, then I can do it with multiple sclerosis!

The two options my nephrologist had to offer me were prednisone therapy or prednisone therapy. So, I chose the lesser of two evils and started the prednisone therapy, which was necessary for the crisis at hand, but I also decided to look for alternative solutions. You and I both know that prednisone can pull us out of an autoimmune crisis, but the price we pay in this treatment is difficult to choose on an ongoing basis. The weight gain (and all of the comments that come with that), mood swings, elevated glucose levels, decreased bone density, impact on the thyroid, eye disease and psychological impact are all a massive cost.

Steroids are also used for M.S. flare-ups, as you have probably already experienced. A percentage of you may find benefit from the ABC (AVONEX®, Betaseron®, Copaxone®) drugs for M.S., but for the rest of us, at this point in time, allopathic medicine can only offer us crisis management. There are more allopathic treatments on the way, but what about fixing the root cause of autoimmune diseases? What would that world look like? At the very least, can we minimize the necessity for crisis intervention with steroids and immuno-suppressants?

In my search for alternative treatments for kidney disease, I came across many fantastic practitioners, who put the kidney disease into remission. So when I was diagnosed with M.S., I used the same practitioners, with greater determination, for my cause of "fixing" it. I may not be at the "fixed" mark, but I feel fantastic and consider it a criminal act to not publish what I have learned for the benefit of patients and physicians who manage multiple sclerosis. Keep in mind, my fixes may not be the same fixes for you, so I encourage you to journey on your own "fix it" path if you are inclined. I will also advise you to have a support system lined up to pick you up when you hit the bumps in your road now and again, and again.

The discussion in this book is in no way a recommendation to "break up" with your neurologist! I see my neurologist every six months and get MRIs regularly to track my progress. If I happen to have a flare up, I still call my neurologist. Again, I am responsible about keeping him alerted to what I am doing and I trust him to slap me upside the head if ever necessary. I pass my test results around to all of my practitioners and keep them informed of my progress. I consider myself responsible for my health and I am the C.E.O. of my health care corporation. Communication with all of my practitioners is a major component in my success.

In addition to having alternative medical care already in place due to my kidney disease, I had a powerful cognitive shift that further adjusted my approach to my health. I was sitting in the Self Expression and Leadership Program of Landmark Education and I realized that after the onset of my kidney disease and M.S., much of my suffering was due to the fact that I had to change my life to manage my health. I stopped going to dance classes and stopped going out with friends because I was too tired. My "to do" list became shorter and shorter and I convinced myself I had to rest all of the time. After working all day, I sometimes had only enough energy to run one errand in the evening and if I attempted two errands, forget it. I did not have the energy to do the things I used to enjoy, and I did not have the money for those things because all of my money was dumped into my health care. How could I live rest of my life bored, limited and resting all the time? Instead of managing my "to do" list to accommodate my health issues, I decided to manage my health to facilitate the "to do" list I desired.

Throughout this publication I will let you know what I did, the approach I took and which products and nutritional supplements I use. I would like to be clear that I have not received any compensation for making these recommendations. These products work for me, but feel free to explore equivalent substitutes that suit your tastes, smells and budgets. I will keep things to the point and underline the items to pay attention to if you want to skip the corresponding babble.

Where possible, I will include references to scientific publications offering support to the discussed remedies. I accessed many of the publications at http://www.ncbi.nlm.nih.gov. This website is a great resource for you to access the articles I discuss in this publication, as well as for additional research you may wish to conduct.

Feel free to pick and choose the remedies that suit you in this publication, don't pick anything, borrow what you like based on your symptoms, make them your own, be happy, be healthy, and take charge.

THE BASIC SCIENCE OF MULTIPLE SCLEROSIS

Your neurologist most likely covered the scientific aspects of your multiple sclerosis, but I want to give you an extremely broad overview of what is happening in your head and spine.

Demyelination and inflammation are major components of our multiple sclerosis. In the inflammatory process, components called macrophages, which are phagocytic mononuclear leukocytes found in tissues, engulf solid particles from their surroundings. In our M.S., macrophages phagocytize (engulf) the myelin sheath surrounding oligodendrocytes (nerves), which further stimulates an immune response. The engulfment of myelin by the macrophage is called demyelination.

Why do we need myelin around our nerves? The myelin sheath "...greatly increases the rate at which an axon can conduct an action potential. So, demyelination will result in the decrease or loss of nerve impulses." [2] It is from this demyelination that we experience symptoms ranging from tingling in our hands and feet to paralysis because our nerves cannot conduct action potentials properly.

After demyelination, either the nerve will remyelinate or it will remain demyelinated. The treatments I will discuss are tools that I have found to reduce inflammation, prevent demyelination and to provide the body with the metabolites necessary for remyelination.

---

[2] Alberts B., Johnson A., Lewis J., Raff M., Roberts K. and Walter P. The molecular biology of the cell. Fourth edition. Garland Science, New York, NY. 2002. P 641.

FIND A CHINESE HERBALIST OR AYURVEDIC DOCTOR

The first thing I did was to find an Ayurvedic doctor. Ayurveda is a form of medicine that originated in India 5,000 years ago. For the western audience, it is difficult to understand and accept Ayurveda as a valid form of medicine. Ayurvedic medicine is a codified science taught in four-year medical schools in the same manner as allopathy (western medicine). Many people do not trust this form of medicine because the treatments have not been plugged and chugged through U.S. universities and approved by the F.D.A. I tend to take the approach that 5,000 years of experiential data far outweighs any pharmaceutical company's twelve-week clinical trial. This form of treatment has been tried, tested and modified for centuries. The approach in Ayurvedic medicine is to treat the cause of a disease using herbal medicines, dietary changes and lifestyle changes. Chinese medicine was derived from Ayurvedic medicine and takes the same approach to healing.

The Maharishi Ayurvedic establishment has centers around the world, although they are quite pricey. I went to The Raj in Iowa for a few days and learned about diet, circadian rhythms and the basics of Ayurvedic science.

The physician instructed me drink a tea every day having manjista, gulunch, and gokru. I boil these items in two quarts of water for 10 minutes and cool it to room temperature. Then, I sip this tea throughout the day. I recently added turmeric and coriander seeds to this recipe. After three weeks of taking this, I noticed a difference in all of my autoimmune conditions, starting with the eczema on my hands completely clearing and remaining in remission. Manjista in particular is beneficial for autoimmune diseases and turmeric is a potent anti-inflammatory agent.

Please do not just leap in and take the same things that I take. *Your* body may require different herbs, so you should consult with an Ayurvedic physician for the best formula for you. You can find a practitioner at www.mapi.com. The website www.theraj.com has case studies of the benefits of this practice for multiple sclerosis patients. If you do not wish to travel to their centers, try to locate a practitioner near to you through Google™ or through friends and family. I have tried Ayurvedic practitioners, and Chinese herbalists, trained in the Asia and America, and highly recommend using physicians that are native to India and trained there. The training is better and more complete than western trained doctors and I have found the treatments to be more effective. At the very least, be cautious not to go to practitioners trained through short courses.

I have been fortunate to be in the care of the former physician to the Dalai Lama, Dr. Yeshi Dhonden. His clinic is in India but he comes to the U.S. about twice a year. I fly to wherever he is in the U.S. for my appointments and go to extreme efforts for his care. It is well worth the effort as Dr. Dhonden was greatly responsible for my kidney disease going into remission and his medicines for M.S. have been extremely effective for me as well. I also have a local Ayurvedic physician for any care I may need in between my appointments with my primary Ayurvedic care provider. Chinese medicine is just as beneficial and again, I recommend a practitioner native to Asia.

Be prepared for many dietary restrictions, which are difficult to adhere to, but will benefit you in the long run. I am restricted from having coffee, all melons, poultry, pork, bell peppers, carrots, radishes, raw onions, pineapples, sesame seeds, poppy seeds, pickles, mangos (this one is painful), kiwis and the list goes on. Again, do not take on these same dietary restrictions, because each person will have different restrictions. I am quite disciplined in this regard. I think to myself, "I would rather have my health than my mangos."

VITAMIN D SUPPLEMENTATION

These days, the buzz in the world of multiple sclerosis is about the role of vitamin D_3 as it relates to M.S. It has long been known that the occurrence of multiple sclerosis is mapped to colder climates, such as the northern parts of North America, Western Europe and the like. It is known that the exposure to sunlight is less in these areas due to the colder climates, and therefore the individuals in these areas may not have the same levels of vitamin D as individuals in other areas where the climate is more conducive to exposure to sunlight. A study published by Wingerchuck et al. entitled "A pilot study of oral calcitriol (1,25-dihydroxyvitamin D3) for relapsing–remitting multiple sclerosis" discusses a suggested link between vitamin D deficiency and increased occurrence of multiple sclerosis. In this study, 15 M.S. patients received vitamin D_3 supplementation. These patients were evaluated on this treatment and continued being monitored after discontinuation. The study showed improvement/stabilization of multiple sclerosis on the treatment, and a worsening of symptoms after discontinuation. [3]

There are a couple of research studies that you can take into your doctor's office as a reference for a discussion on vitamin D supplementation. Both of these studies support the Wingerchuck study indicating a reduction of multiple sclerosis symptoms with vitamin D supplementation, and furthering the discussion with clinical recommendations such as dosage and monitoring of serum levels of vitamin D. The first article is entitled "Safety of vitamin D3 in adults with multiple sclerosis" by Kimball et al. This study determined doses of vitamin D_3 that are therapeutically effective as well as tolerable. The

---

[3] Wingerchuk, D.M, Lesaux, J, Rice, G.P.A., Kremenchutzky, M., Ebers, G. C. A pilot study of oral calcitriol (1,25-dihydroxyvitamin D3) for relapsing–remitting multiple sclerosis. J Neurol Neurosurg Psychiatry. 2005;76:1294–1296.

tolerability was determined by increasing the serum levels of 25-hydroxyvitamin D, while not causing hypercalcemia. In this study, the levels of vitamin D were increased to 386 +/- 157 nmol/L, which actually decreased the enhancing lesions on MRIs. It was also found that the amount of 25-hydroxyvitamin D in the serum was about twice the amount of the top level of the presently accepted normal range, without causing hypercalcemia or hypercalciuria. [4]

The second article is entitled "Use of Vitamin D in Clinical Practice" by Cannell et al. This study found that vitamin D supplementation reduces ALL causes of mortality and urges prompt assessment of vitamin D levels in patients across the board. This study recommends treating healthy patients with 2,000 to 7,000 IUs a day to maintain year-round levels of serum 25-hydroxyvitamin D at about 40-70 ng/mL. However, for patients with serious illnesses, including multiple sclerosis, the year-round levels of

---

[4] Kimball, S. M., Ursell, M.R. Ursell, O'Conner, P., and Vieth, R. Safety of vitamin D3 in adults with multiple sclerosis. Am J Clin Nutr. 2007;86:645–51.

serum 25-hydroxyvitamin D should be maintained at 55-70 ng/mL.[5]

You may note the discrepancy in the recommended serum levels of 25-hydroxyvitamin D between Kimball et al. and Cannell et al. This is why I suggest that you take these articles in to your doctor's office to discuss these findings. These recommendations are very recent, and further studies are being conducted as I type, so by the time you get to your doctor's office, there may be more updated clinical recommendations. If you do begin vitamin D supplementation, don't forget to be regularly monitored for hypercalcemia and hypercalciuria.

My serum 25-hydroxyvitamin D was 9 ng/mL, which is deficient. After supplementation, my levels are at about 73 ng/mL and I am experiencing greatly reduced symptoms.

---

[5] Cannell, J.J. and Hollis, B.W. Use of Vitamin D in Clinical Practice. Alternative Medicine Review. 2008;13(1);6-20.

NUTRITIONAL SUPPLEMENTS

I have found a key component in remyelinating my nerves is to provide my body with all of the components in the myelin sheath so that when my body makes the attempt to repair the myelin, it has the tools to do so.

The myelin sheath is made of sphingomeyelin, phosphatidylethanolamine, phosphotidlyserine, cholesterol, glycolipids and other components. At the onset of my M.S., my local Ayurvedic physician recommended a combination of several supplements, which would provide all of the building blocks needed to synthesize all of the above mentioned components. These include a <u>vegetarian amino acid powder mixture, a 3-6-9- omega liquid oil and a fiber mixture all stirred in water.</u> You can combine these items in juice or water, although I use water because my orange juice is sacred and making sludge out of it is sacrilegious in my world. In a cup of water, I mix two heaping teaspoons (not the measuring tsp., but the cutlery tsp.) of the amino acid powder, two heaping teaspoons of the fiber and two tablespoons of the oil. Upon mixing, the consistency is thick and like sludge. With the sludge, I take 1,300 mg of Evening Primrose Oil, which is a source of linoleic acid, and 1,000 mg of ginger in capsule form, which is a good anti-inflammatory agent.

The fiber mix I used is called Superfood Supplement, Omega 3 Basic®, Original, Master Nutrient Formula™. It is manufactured by Designing Health, Inc. (800-774-7387 and the website is www.designinghealth.com).

Vegetarian Protein Booster made by Naturade. This comes with soy or soy free and is distributed by Naturade, Inc., 14370 Myford Rd., Irvine CA, 92606. You can also find them at www.naturade.com. If you are hypothyroid, please use the soy free version.

The Essential Balance Oil is from Omega Nutrition (866-661-FLAX, www.omeganutrition.com).

Evening Primrose Oil is organic and hexane free from Spectrum Organic Products, Inc., (800-995-2705, www.spectrumorganic.com).

I take "the sludge" in the morning, a minimum of 30 minutes before breakfast, or any other consumption. By the way, this is rock star fiber you have in this mixture. It will help your M.S. related constipation. Yeah! If you are not inclined to do anything else that I suggest in this publication, this supplementation is what I feel is most important.

GET YOUR THYROID CHECKED

As many of you already know, people with one autoimmune condition tend to be prone to a plurality of autoimmune conditions. My autoimmune conditions started with a small patch of psoriasis on my head when I was 10 years old, then progressed to asthma when I was 15, then Stein-Leventhal Syndrome in high school, then focal segmental glomerulosclerosis and multiple sclerosis.

A very common problem affecting about 10-15% of women in the U.S. is Hashimoto thyroiditis. Many women are undiagnosed with this condition because in typical screening, the thyroid panel only tests TSH, Free T4 and T3 uptake. I intuitively kept bugging my doctor to check my thyroid because I was fatigued, gaining weight and my hair was falling out for years. But, the thyroid values were always in the normal range, so I was considered to have normal thyroid function.

I found my way back to the University of Wisconsin Hospital and Clinics where my physician's first instinct in treating my exercise-induced anaphylaxis was to check the titer of my thyroid peroxidase antibodies. The test results showed that the anti-thyroid antibodies were greater than 35 times the normal range. The physician correlated this high titer to my urticaria and anaphylaxis and my Ayurvedic physician also correlated this to my asthma and hives. The levothyroxine therapy was ineffective in reducing the antibody titer, so I began additional Ayurvedic treatment for this. After one year, the antibody titer has decreased to 2.5 times greater than the high end of the normal range.

I also began taking a thyroid balancing herbal formula made by GAIA Herb, Inc. in Brevard, North Carolina. The product name is Liquid Phyto-Caps "Thyroid Support." This supplement contains L-tyrosine, Schizandra berry, Coleus root, Kelp fronds, Ashwagandha and Bladderwrack fronds. I noticed a remarkable improvement in my emotive stability within one week of starting this supplement and my hair also stopped falling out. You can find a distributor at www.gaiaherbs.com. Please remember, what works for me may not work for you. Again, it is best to consult your herbalist and/or physician when adding or subtracting items from your health care system.

A study authored by M. Fernandez, et al. entitled "Thyroid hormone administration enhances remyelination of chronic demyelinating inflammatory disease," showed that thyroid hormone enhanced and accelerated remyelination in rats by increasing levels of platelet derived growth factor receptor when administered in acute phases of disease.[6] [7] This further restored normal levels of myelin basic protein mRNA and protein. In addition, thyroid hormone has been found to be neuroprotective.

It seems to be important to address thyroid health in M.S. patients, and it is unfortunate that this condition remains undiagnosed in many individuals. Treating my thyroid has relieved the fatigue I previously attributed to M.S. I do not intend to negate the fatigue aspect of my M.S., but I think it was compounded by the thyroid disease.

If you find that you are hypothyroid, or if your thyroid panel values are in the normal ranges but you have a high antibody titer, remember to stay away from soy products.

---

[6] Fernandez M., Giuliani A, Pirondi S, D'Intino G, Giardino L, Aloe L, Levi-Montalcini R and Calza L. Thyroid hormone administration enhances remyelination of chronic demyelinating inflammatory disease. Proc Natl Acad Sci U.S.A., 2004 Nov 16; 101(46):16363-8. Epub 2004 Nov 8.

[7] Calza L, Fernandez M, Giuliani A, D'Intino G, Pirondi S, Sivilia S, Paradisi M, Desordi N and Giardino L. Thyroid Hormone and remyelination in adult central nervous system: a lesson from an inflammatory demyelinating disease. Brain Res Brain Rex Rev. 2005, Apr; 48(2):339-46. Epub. 2005, Jan 26.

PHOSPHOROUS

One of my friends, an allopathic physician and a homeopathic physician, was helping me along with my health issues. When my M.S. popped up, he immediately recommended taking phosphorous. He said it would provide significant relief. So, I took it on faith.

Then a year later, I took a trip to India and saw this friend again. He said I had not been taking the right dose and he increased my dose from of phosphorous from 30C to 200C.

Time went on and one day I sat down to check out the latest on remyelination on PubMed at http://www.ncbi.nlm.nih.gov. I found that the phosphorylation of tyrosine had been found to be a key factor in myelin formation.[8] Tyrosine is in the amino acid powder and some thyroid supplements. Phosphorylation is known as a post-translational modification of proteins, meaning that phosphorous will attach to a protein after it has been synthesized to further its activity. Therefore, it is a good idea to make sure you have enough phosphorous in your diet or through supplements.

It excites me that the ancient medicines of homeopathy and Ayurveda are all coming together with current research in the U.S. and gaining validity. So, pick up some phosphorous the next time you are at your homeopathic pharmacy. It is probably a good idea to find a homeopathic physician for dosages and a treatment plan suited to you.

[8] Harroch, Sheila et al. A critical role for the protein tyrosine phosphatase receptor type Z in functional recovery from demyelination lesions. Nature Genetics. Published online. 30 September 2002

REDUCE HEAT EXPOSURE, BETTER YET, SWING THE OTHER WAY

Exposure to heat is one of the most common triggers of an M.S. flare up. Whether it is solar or indoor heat, it is crucial to manage exposure on a daily basis. An Internet-based survey was conducted with 2,529 anonymous participants to explore the experiences that affect patients with M.S.[9] High stress levels, high temperatures and viral infections were reported to be common triggers. For me, temperature is HUGE!

It is a good idea to try to deduce which temperature range is optimal for you. I know that I start to feel "M.S.-ey" if I am in temperatures above 72 degrees F. You will have your own temperature ranges that

[9] Simmons RD, Ponsonby, AL, Van Der Mei, I A.F., Sheridan P. Multiple Sclerosis. Publisher: Hodder Arnold Journals. Volume 10, Number 2, 1 April 2004, pp. 202-211(10).

trigger your symptoms. Take some time to figure that out and then launch into managing your temperature exposure. This part may be a hassle because it requires that you think ten steps ahead of yourself, but it is well worth the effort. Not only do I reduce heat exposure, I take every opportunity to cool my body as I find this helps my symptoms.

The first thing I do every morning is to take a freezing cold shower. If I start to feel M.S.-ey, we all can feel it coming on, I hop in a cold shower and I feel better instantly. Tepid or lukewarm water does not work for me, but it may work for you. I got that hot tip from an amazing woman who has had M.S. for 32 years, is the C.E.O. of two corporations and plays tennis every day.

If you live in a place that is hot all year round, move north. Hanging out in L.A. for a job, while you are barely surviving due to the heat, is not worth it.

If you live in a place with four seasons and you have a summer to survive, get a remote car starter installed. In the summer keep your car A.C. set to "cold" and start your car a few minutes before you have to sit in it. The remote starters cost a few hundred bucks, but it is well worth cooling your car to spare you the few minutes of smoldering heat.

Ask your place of employment, school or anywhere you spend time regularly, to provide accommodations for temperature. I work closely with my graduate school and place of employment to maintain the temperature between 68 and 70 degrees F. This is a "reasonable accommodation" in most buildings as provided by the Americans with Disabilities Act, with some exceptions.

Think ahead. If you are going to the theater, call ahead and ask what their temperature settings are. If you are riding in a friend's car to go shopping, ask if she would mind keeping the heat in the car on the lower side. If you are going to Yoga class, ask them at what temperature they keep the room. Skip the sauna-like Bikram yoga. Don't flirt with the rental car hunk in the hot summer sun. If you ever find yourself in a room that is too hot, politely excuse yourself and get somewhere cooler immediately.

Buy sunhats to suit your personality and wear them without fail when it is sunny outside.

Apply ice packs immediately if you start to feel like you have been exposed to heat. Carry those blue bags that you can get at any drug store to fill with ice. Ziploc® bags are just as easy to carry around in your purse. I was in LaGuardia airport, the terminal was not air-conditioned and it was 90 degrees F outside. I pulled out my Ziploc® bag and asked one of the places in the food court if I could buy ice from them. They filled my bag, took a buck and saved the day. You can also carry the cold packs that you squeeze to activate by chemical reaction. I buy a case at a time of these and carry a couple of them with me wherever I go.

Ask your employer if you can work from home when the weather is too warm to go outside. I have been blessed with great employers in this regard and I am able to work from home when necessary.

If you have a job that will not allow for this, then sit down with your employer to see what kind of accommodations can be made to help you make it through the summer or any other day that may be too warm for you. If you are hesitant to disclose your M.S. to your employer, which is a very valid hesitation, brainstorm any accommodations you can make on your own. Purchase a fan or a cooler for your desk or leave a few minutes earlier in the morning so you can get a closer parking spot at work.

If it is too hot for you to go outside, get groceries delivered from an internet delivery service. You can also call your local grocery store to see if they can deliver groceries if you don't have any internet based services in your area. If you just explain the situation and ask politely for a delivery, you will be pleasantly surprised at the humanity that will receive you. Once, I needed a printer cartridge because I was working from home and was facing deadlines, for which I needed to print. Ack! I called Staples and asked the manager if they had any delivery service. No, of course not, and I did not have time to place an internet order and wait a few days for delivery. After I explained my situation to this gentleman, I found that he was a completely gracious soul and he ran the cartridge over to my house to help me get through my deadlines. You will find such angels everywhere.

Just this past year, I got over my pride and got a temporary handicap sticker for my car to use in the summertime. This allows me to park closer to doors and to limit my heat exposure even further. Because many cities are cracking down on the abuse of handicap parking permits, and given that I am still able bodied, I carry a letter from my physician in my purse explaining my condition and the exacerbation of M.S. from heat exposure.

It is sad, but your sunbathing days are over. I know some of you are still sunbathing. The only thing to do is KNOCK IT OFF!

I carry around a portable thermometer that I purchased from REI. My sister considers this obsessive behavior. I consider it being responsible.

Don't stand in front of the oven door when you pull out a batch of cookies, do ask your hair dresser to wash your hair with cold water, do use hair dryers on the cool setting, don't cook with all four burners active and ask to be moved in a restaurant that seats you under a heating vent. Be extremely diligent and responsible for yourself when it comes to heat.

CHERRIES FOR INFLAMMATION

My personal journey through Multiple Sclerosis is complicated by kidney disease, so I have to be particularly careful not to take any drugs that would impact my kidneys. Drugs metabolized by the kidneys and anti-inflammatory medicine like ibuprofen, naproxen sodium, and the like, are all forbidden for me. I stumbled across a blurb in an issue of *The Bottom Line*, indicating cherries have anti-inflammatory properties. Cherries in any form apparently have this effect. I gave it a try considering I could not take other forms of anti-inflammatories and I found cherries to be quite effective in managing my inflammation.

I stock up on bags and bags of dried cherries. I keep some at work, some in my bag and a nice big stash at home. About 20 cherries seem to provide relief for my headaches and M.S.-ey feelings. Cherries, in combination with an ice pack on my head and a nap help even more.

As previously mentioned, inflammation accompanies demyelination because the myelin is engulfed by macrophages and the macrophages secrete inflammatory mediators. In *Biochemical Pharmacology*, it was reported that compounds called flavanoids actually decrease the amount of myelin that is phagocytized by the macrophages.[10] The three most effective flavanoids for this are leteolin, quercetin and fisetin. Well folks, cherries are loaded with quercetin. So eat tons of cherries! I tend to buy organic dried cherries, which is tough on the wallet, but conventionally grown cherries will also do.

There are a few more berries that are great source of quercetin including blackcurrants, lingonberries and bilberries. I do not know the relative amounts

---

[10] Hendriks, J, de Vries H.E., van der Pol S.M.A., van den Berg T.K., van Tol E.A.F. and Dijkstra C.D. Flavanoids inhibit myelin phagocytosis by macrophages; a structure-activity relationship study. Biochemical Pharmacology, Volume 65, Issue 5, 1 March 2003, Pages 877-885.

of these flavanoids in these various berries, but it may be worth some investigation if you have the time. You may also buy quercetin in the form of pills. It is not a bad idea to line up all of these different forms and see which one works best for you. I did not find the pills to be very effective for me, but you may like them better. Other sources of quercetin are apple skins, onions, raspberries, citrus fruits, broccoli, leafy greens and green and black tea.

There are also many herbs and spices that are potent anti-inflammatory agents such as basil, cardamom, cilantro, cinnamon, clove, ginger, parsley and turmeric. Use these every day if you can. These herbs and spices should probably be used by people with elevated glucose levels, so as not to jeopardize glucose control by eating cherries and other fruits. Again, consult with your physician on such issues.

HYPNOTHERAPY

Grasping at straws, when I was managing my kidney disease, I began hypnotherapy once a week to improve my symptoms. I noted a decrease in proteinurea as a regular occurrence after my hypnosis sessions. I was pleased with the relaxation it provided and the improvement of symptoms. After the M.S. diagnosis, my fantastic hypnotherapist added healing suggestions for this condition. When I am feeling M.S.-ey, after a single session, I feel a significant reduction in pain and discomfort, which I normally experience in my head. Although this treatment has not been researched at length, there are case reports indicating an improvement in the symptoms of M.S. patients after hypnosis sessions.

In a case report authored by H. Sutcher, this preliminary report suggests that hypnosis can facilitate healing in M.S. patients.[11] The report tracked three patients with multiple sclerosis, one who was wheelchair bound, another experienced trouble with balance but otherwise minimal symptoms and a third with pain in her right leg. All three showed immediate improvement or displacement of symptoms with hypnosis.

I highly recommend this form of treatment for relief of symptoms as a supplement to your health care. I typically experience an immediate improvement of my symptoms after a session. The exceptions arise when I am excessively stressed in other areas of my life and have difficulty relaxing during the session. A major benefit to this form of treatment is that there are absolutely no negative side effects. You are not ingesting any food, drug or supplement, making this a no lose treatment option. A health psychologist in your area can provide this treatment. If your insurance does not cover this therapy, I suggest learning how to do self-hypnosis.

---

[11] Sutcher H. Hypnosis as adjunctive therapy for multiple sclerosis: a progress report. Am J Clin Hypn. 1997 Apr; 39(4):283-90.

THE EXTRA MILE

There are several other practices I do regularly. There is not much data available to support the prevention of demyelination or enhancement of remyelination through these practices, but these are things I do that make me feel physically and emotionally better so I continue to do so.

The first is, I purchase organic foods. I know this can be tough on the wallet, but I am clear that ingesting pesticide-laden food is not good for my health. If it is not possible for you to purchase organic versions of all of your groceries, at least try to purchase organic eggs, milk and produce because it is not possible to wash pesticides off many items such as berries and leafy greens.

I get a chiropractic adjustment every two weeks along with a massage. I noticed some pain reduction in my back when I began this care. Your insurance may cover these services due to your condition. If your neurologist can prescribe physical therapy, there is usually a massage therapist working in conjunction with physical therapists and this might be an avenue for coverage for the massage.

Dance /Movement Therapy is a little known practice from which I have received great emotional and physical benefit. Dance/movement therapy was founded on the principle that a vital connection exists between personality and the way in which a person moves his/her body. Through this therapy, changes in movement affect the emotional and physical health of an individual. Research is currently being performed on the neurological impact of dance/movement therapy and the formation of new neural connections. The benefits I received from this type of therapy were improved balance, a reduction in dizziness and an experience of greater connectivity throughout my body. I am also a

Certified Movement Analyst and have correlated my movement and posture to my symptoms, in particular dizziness. To find a practitioner, contact the American Dance Therapy Association (ADTA) at (410) 997-4040 or their website is www.adta.org. In addition, the National M.S. Society website has information and workshops available for M.S. patients.

I also schedule a Rolfing appointment once a month or so. This tends to cost about twice as much as a deep tissue massage, but I receive significant relief in pain. A certified Rolfer repositions bone and muscles to structurally reintegrate your body from being off balance. You can find a practitioner at www.rolf.org.

Don't forget to take care of your mind as well as your body. Openly communicate with people you trust if you are depressed due to your condition. If you are not comfortable opening up to the people in your life then consider counseling, support groups or on-line support. Individuals diagnosed with M.S.

frequently experience moderate to severe depression. Please do not neglect these issues, communication and/or counseling can help you navigate through these feelings and hopefully bring you to a place of acceptance and possibly even power!

Pamper your circadian clock. I have found it most important to go to sleep by 10 p.m. to make it through my days. Your Ayurvedic doctor can help you understand your circadian rhythms and tell you when the best times are to eat, sleep and exercise.

Lastly, I highly recommend finding a neurologist that supports you in pursuing alternative avenues to healing. Or at least, find a doctor that will just roll her eyes and let you continue on your way. My neurologist was the fourth I "interviewed" for the job (Doc, I bet you didn't know that.). I value intelligent and compassionate physicians along with an open mind. I literally interview physicians on the phone before I make an appointment. I ask them about their practice, their approach to their patients and opinions on alternative medicine. I truly believe that a physician who is committed to your well-being will acknowledge the limitations of his/her training and realize that there are tools available that were not taught in medical school. I think it is very important to have a neurologist caring for you, but if he or she is not seeing beyond the ABC drugs or steroids, then it might not be a bad idea to break up with him or her and find a different neurologist who will support you in feeling better holistically.

A DAY IN THE LIFE OF…

Some of you may be a bit overwhelmed reading all of the things I do, so I am going to take you through one of my typical days. This schedule is not inflexible and there are always variations here and there. I have increased my level of discipline in hopes of sticking to this schedule as best as I can. I am clear that sometimes I may come across as rigid, but averting disability is of utmost importance for me. I highly recommend being in the frame of mind of "I'll do whatever it takes, even if that means ________(you fill in the blank)."

Here is how my average day goes:

> 5:30 AM to 6:00 AM: Wake up and take my first dose of Ayurvedic medicine and exercise for one hour.

6:30 AM: Take the protein/fiber/oil sludge with evening primrose oil and ginger capsules. Begin boiling my Ayurvedic tea that I sip for the day and hop in the shower. By the time I am out of the shower, the tea has been boiling for about 10 minutes. Turn off heat and let cool to room temperature and put it in a thermos to take to work.

7:15 AM: With breakfast I have a cup of black tea with crushed cardamom pods, fennel seeds and ginger, which have anti-inflammatory properties.

9:00 AM: Phosphorous dose.

10:30 AM: Thyroid supplement.

12:00 PM: Lunch, with 50,000 IU vitamin D twice a week. Your digestive enzymes are highest around noon for the day, so it is best to eat your biggest meal now.

1:00 or 1:30 PM: Second dose of Ayurvedic medicine.

4:00 PM: Third dose of Ayurvedic medicine.

6:00 PM: Thyroid supplement.

9:00 PM: Phones get shut off. Everyone knows not to call me after 9 PM, even when I am feeling fine. Take fourth dose of Ayurvedic medicine.

9:30 PM – 10:00 PM: Bedtime.

Anytime during the day if I feel the need, I ice my head and have a few dried cherries. I also have a couple of cups of green tea during the workday.

I schedule hypnotherapy once or twice a week right after work.

The chiropractor and massage are every other Saturday morning and the Rolfing is once a month.

I have my heat management system in place by having my office preset to 68 degrees F. My university monitors and cools the room temperature of my lecture halls when I am on campus. I also have cold packs and sunhats with me to avoid or manage any heat exposure.

If that schedule came across as daunting, don't be discouraged. I keep all of medicines for the day on my desk at work, and the doses in the morning and night are easy to remember. Give yourself some time to adjust if you are going to incorporate some of these into your routine. Of course there are days when I sleep late, space out, forget to take something, am in a movie or out clubbing. Give yourself the leeway to enjoy life, but eventually return to your schedule so you can regain and maintain your health.

KNOW YOUR RIGHTS

I highly recommend that you familiarize yourself with the Americans with Disabilities Act at www.eeoc.gov. Some employers are resistant to providing reasonable accommodations to assist you through any disabilities you may have or wish to prevent. Always document any conversation or situation related to your health. This includes positive and supportive conversations, as well as ones that are not accommodating or that make you uncomfortable. Try not to look for trouble where there isn't any, but the documentation will serve you if you ever find yourself in a bind.

Some states have organizations designed to assist you in situations where you require legal assistance, direction in obtaining disability accommodations or if you feel that you are being discriminated against.

One example of such an organization is Equip For Equality (www.equipforequality.org). The staff and attorneys at these organizations are specifically trained to advise and assist you through these circumstances.

Scope out affordable attorneys in advance so if you ever face discrimination, you have a system in place to protect and defend your rights to work and maneuver through life. Pre-paid legal services may make you feel more secure if the need arises in the future (http://www.prepaidlegal.com).

IMPORTANT NOTICE

This publication does not provide healthcare advice. Consult your physician before starting any nutritional supplement program.

The statements made about the effects of the dietary supplements in publication have not been evaluated by the Food and Drug Administration. Dietary and nutritional supplements are intended for special dietary use. They are not intended for use in the treatment, cure, prevention or mitigation of any disease or disorder. They are intended to be used as part of an overall healthy lifestyle program that includes proper diet and exercise. Only your doctor can properly diagnose and treat any disease or disorder. Before starting to use any nutritional supplement, it is important to check with your doctor.

You should consult with your physician before starting the disclosed nutritional supplements and lifestyle suggestions. Regular exercise and proper nutrition are essential to achieving your desired physique and level of fitness and health. There are no typical results.

It is important to read and follow all label directions carefully. The discussed supplements are not intended for children or for pregnant or lactating women. Not all supplements are appropriate for everyone. In any case, it is prudent for those who have not been taking nutritional supplements to gradually increase their daily dosage to reach the desired amount after consulting a physician and it is important to be followed by a regular physician during the course of any change in diet, lifestyle and supplementation.

The products, information, services and other content provided, including without limitation any products, information, services and other content provided on any Linked Site, are provided for informational purposes only to facilitate discussions with your physician or other healthcare professional regarding treatment options.

The information provided in this publication and on any Linked Sites, including without limitation information relating to medical and health conditions, products and treatments, is often provided in summary or aggregate form. It is not intended as a substitute for advice from your healthcare professional, or any information contained on or in any product label or packaging.

You should not use the information or services for diagnosis or treatment of any health issue or for prescription of any medication or other treatment. You should always speak with your healthcare professional, and carefully read all information provided by the manufacturer of a product and on or in any product label or packaging, before using any medication or nutritional, herbal or homeopathic product, before starting any diet or exercise program or before adopting any treatment for a health problem. Each person is different, and the way you react to a particular product may be significantly different from the way other people react to such product. You should also consult your physician or healthcare professional regarding any interactions between any medication you are currently taking and nutritional supplements.

You are advised that other sites on the Internet, including without limitation Linked Sites, might contain material or information that some people may find offensive or inappropriate; or that is inaccurate, untrue, misleading or deceptive; or that is defamatory, libelous, infringing of others' rights or otherwise unlawful. The author expressly disclaims any responsibility for the content, legality, decency or accuracy of any information, and for any products and services, that appear on any Linked Site.

Again, if you are considering adding nutritional supplements to your diet, please consult your physician. He or she can provide valuable information about any possible drug interactions and help you make an informed choice about whether the supplement you're considering fits your individual health needs.

END NOTES

[1] Hirshberg, C. & Barasch, M. I. Remarkable Recovery. Riverhead Books, published by the Berkley Publishing Group, New York, NY. (1995).

[2] Alberts B., Johnson A., Lewis J., Raff M., Roberts K. and Walter P. The molecular biology of the cell. Fourth edition. Garland Science, New York, NY. 2002. P 641.

[3] Wingerchuk, D.M, Lesaux, J, Rice, G.P.A., Kremenchutzky, M., Ebers, G. C. A pilot study of oral calcitriol (1,25-dihydroxyvitamin D3) for relapsing–remitting multiple sclerosis. J Neurol Neurosurg Psychiatry. 2005;76:1294–1296.

[4] Kimball, S. M., Ursell, M.R. Ursell, O'Conner, P., and Vieth, R. Safety of vitamin D3 in adults with multiple sclerosis. Am J Clin Nutr. 2007;86:645–51.

[5] Cannell, J.J. and Hollis, B.W. Use of Vitamin D in Clinical Practice. Alternative Medicine Review. 2008;13(1);6-20.

[6] Fernandez M., Giuliani A, Pirondi S, D'Intino G, Giardino L, Aloe L, Levi-Montalcini R and Calza L. Thyroid hormone administration enhances remyelination of chronic demyelinating inflammatory disease. Proc

Natl Acad Sci U.S.A., 2004 Nov 16; 101(46):16363-8. Epub 2004 Nov 8.

[7] Calza L, Fernandez M, Giuliani A, D'Intino G, Pirondi S, Sivilia S, Paradisi M, Desordi N and Giardino L. Thyroid Hormone and remyelination in adult central nervous system: a lesson from an inflammatory demyelinating disease. Brain Res Brain Rex Rev. 2005, Apr; 48(2):339-46. Epub. 2005, Jan 26.

[8] Harroch, Sheila et al. A critical role for the protein tyrosine phosphatase receptor type Z in functional recovery from demyelination lesions. Nature Genetics. Published online. 30 September 2002.

[9] Simmons RD, Ponsonby, AL, Van Der Mei, I A.F., Sheridan P. Multiple Sclerosis. Publisher: Hodder Arnold Journals. Volume 10, Number 2, 1 April 2004, pp. 202-211(10).

[10] Hendriks, J, de Vries H.E., van der Pol S.M.A., van den Berg T.K., van Tol E.A.F. and Dijkstra C.D. Flavanoids inhibit myelin phagocytosis by macrophages; a structure-activity relationship study. Biochemical Pharmacology, Volume 65, Issue 5, 1 March 2003, Pages 877-885.

[11] Sutcher H. Hypnosis as adjunctive therapy for multiple sclerosis: a progress report. Am J Clin Hypn. 1997 Apr; 39(4):283-90.

NOTES

NOTES

ABOUT THE AUTHOR

Reena Arora is a molecular biologist and has a Bachelor of Science degree in Genetics from the University of Wisconsin – Madison. She is currently a graduate student in Cellular and Molecular Biology at the Illinois Institute of Technology. Reena spent many years working as a scientist at Abbott Laboratories and in academic research and development environments.

Reena was diagnosed with multiple sclerosis in 2001 and used to experience frequent flare-ups, which included recurring numbness, tingling, nausea, loss of vision and balance, and the general discomfort that many multiple sclerosis patients experience. Initially she was treated with traditional western approaches, but the symptoms remained, so she searched for treatments that would facilitate better health and functioning.

She employed her understanding of cellular and molecular biology to research the scientific basis of the remedies available through alternative care and eastern medicines. She used this knowledge to create a regimen to manage her multiple sclerosis. By using this system, she is essentially free of the symptoms and remains free of disability.

Reena is currently a full time professional, a part time graduate student and a classical Indian dancer and performer. She is excited to share her system in hopes that her efforts will provide multiple sclerosis patients with tools for better health and vitality.

www.ingramcontent.com/pod-product-compliance
Ingram Content Group UK Ltd.
Pitfield, Milton Keynes, MK11 3LW, UK
UKHW041933190726
13854UKWH00004B/1565